Evaluation of Cut-resistant Sleeves and Fiberglass Fiber Shedding at a Steel Mill

Loren Tapp, MD, MS
Diana Ceballos, MS, PhD
Douglas Wiegand, PhD

I0415805

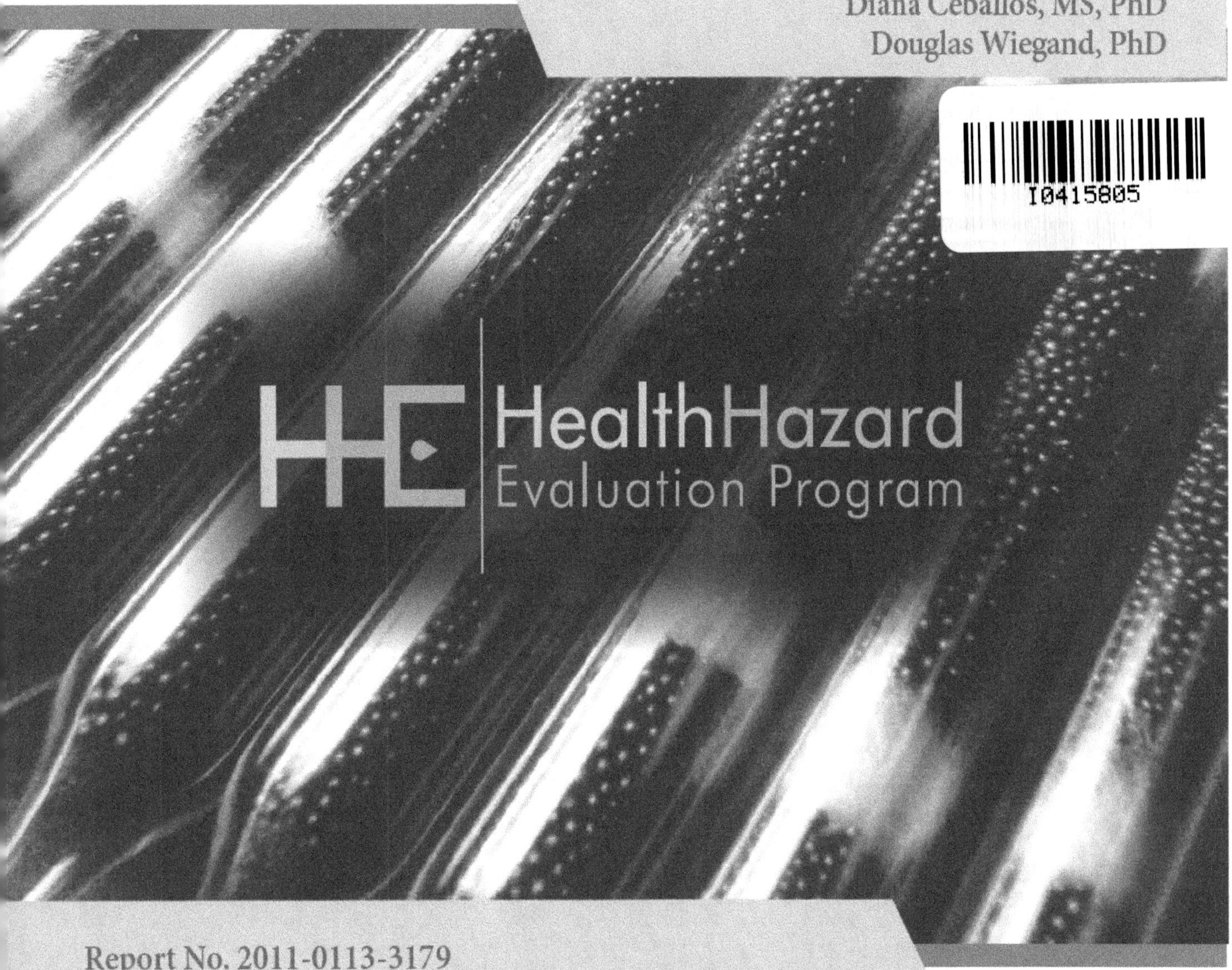

HealthHazard
Evaluation Program

Report No. 2011-0113-3179
May 2013

U.S. Department of Health and Human Services
Centers for Disease Control and Prevention
National Institute for Occupational Safety and Health

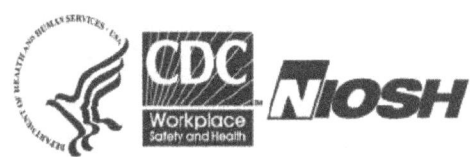

Contents

The cover photo is a close-up image of sorbent tubes, which are used by the HHE Program to measure airborne exposures. This photo is an artistic representation that may not be related to this Health Hazard Evaluation.

Highlights of this Evaluation

The Health Hazard Evaluation Program received a request from a steel mill in Pennsylvania. The employee and union representatives were concerned about skin irritation and possible respiratory problems from fiberglass fibers shedding from their cut-resistant sleeves. They were also concerned about safety and hygiene problems from the required use of these sleeves.

What We Did

- We visited the steel mill in November 2011.

- We toured the plant to see work processes and cut-resistant sleeve use.

- We talked to employees about their work and health concerns.

- We collected tape and vacuum samples from work surfaces, cut-resistant sleeves, and employee clothing and skin.

- We took bulk samples of the new and washed cut-resistant sleeves.

- We identified the type, shape, and size of fibers collected from all of the samples.

- We reviewed the Occupational Safety and Health Administration injury and illness logs and employee medical records.

What We Found

- The size and shape of the fiberglass and Kevlar® fibers shedding from the sleeves make them difficult to inhale into the lungs.

- The composition and size of these fibers make them unlikely to cause any long-term health problems. However, the fiberglass fibers may cause temporary upper respiratory irritation.

> We evaluated cut-resistant sleeves used by steel mill production employees. We found fiberglass fibers on surface, clothing, and skin samples. These fibers may cause temporary skin and upper respiratory irritation, but are unlikely to cause long-term respiratory disease because of their large size. We also found employees were afraid to report injuries and illnesses because of disciplinary action. We recommended providing alternative sleeves for employees with symptoms and improving the safety climate by including employees in decision-making processes.

- Some employees reported numbness and/or pain in the hands or wrists from wearing the sleeves with thick gloves. This is probably due to awkward hand and wrist positions and the extra force needed to grip tools.

- Some employees reported steam burns on their arms or itchy, irritated skin from wearing the cut-resistant sleeves. No employees we interviewed had a rash or burn.

- Employees were concerned about heat stress, poor hygiene practices, and safety hazards related to wearing the sleeves.

What We Found (continued)

- Skin and surface samples contained fiberglass, Kevlar, and cellulose fibers from the cut-resistant sleeves.

- New and washed cut-resistant sleeves had fiberglass bundles with broken fibers and Kevlar fibers that were frayed. These fibers did not have sharp edges.

- The injury and illness logs reported one tenth the number of entries of the U.S. steel industry average.

- Most employees we talked with felt uncomfortable reporting work-related injuries and illnesses or telling their supervisor about their safety and health concerns. They felt that reporting would lead to disciplinary action.

What the Employer Can Do

- Review the policy of requiring cut-resistant sleeve use by all employees.

- Provide a different type of cut-resistant sleeves for employees who have skin irritation, hand pain, or wrist pain from the cut-resistant sleeves they had been wearing.

- Provide new and washed cut-resistant sleeves in more locations that are easy to get to throughout the steel mill, including employee locker rooms.

- Do not allow employees to take cut-resistant sleeves home.

- Keep track of how many times the sleeves have been washed.

- Train employees how to care for, maintain, and dispose of sleeves.

- Check sleeves returned by the laundry service regularly to make sure they are cleaned adequately.

- Include employees and union representatives in discussions and decisions about safety and health procedures and policies. Consider hiring an external safety consultant to aid in improving safety climate in the workplace.

- Encourage employees to report work-related injuries and illnesses as soon as possible.

What Employees Can Do

- Do not take cut-resistant sleeves home.

- Look at sleeves closely before you reuse them and do not use damaged, frayed, or soiled sleeves.

- Tell your supervisor if you have any health or safety concerns, including concerns about wearing the cut-resistant sleeves.

- Report work-related injuries and illnesses to your supervisor as soon as they start.

- Shower and put on clean clothes before you go home.

Mention of any company or product does not constitute endorsement by NIOSH. In addition, citations to websites external to NIOSH do not constitute NIOSH endorsement of the sponsoring organizations or their programs or products. Furthermore, NIOSH is not responsible for the content of these websites. All web addresses referenced in this document were accessible as of the publication date of this report.

Abbreviations

μm	Micrometer
ACGIH®	American Conference of Governmental Industrial Hygienists
BLS	Bureau of Labor Statistics
CFR	Code of Federal Regulations
IARC	International Agency for Research on Cancer
NAICS	North American Industry Classification System
NFPA	National Fire Protection Association
NIOSH	National Institute for Occupational Safety and Health
OEL	Occupational exposure limit
OSHA	Occupational Safety and Health Administration
PEL	Permissible exposure limit
REL	Recommended exposure limit
TLV®	Threshold limit value
TWA	Time-weighted average

Introduction

In May 2011, the National Institute for Occupational Safety and Health (NIOSH) received a health hazard evaluation (HHE) request from employee and union representatives at a steel mill in Pennsylvania. The request concerned skin and upper respiratory irritation and the potential for long-term respiratory disease from the shedding of fiberglass fibers from cut-resistant sleeves. Requestors were also concerned about safety and hygiene issues from the use of these sleeves. During our site visit, we met with union representatives and managers, toured the facility, and confidentially interviewed employees. We took samples of fibers from work surfaces, clothing, and skin of employees, and bulk samples of new sleeves, laundered sleeves, and insulation found at the steel mill. We also reviewed injury and illness logs, material safety data sheets, and medical records. After our site visit, we discussed ergonomic and work stress problems that were identified during the site visit with a NIOSH ergonomist and a NIOSH behavioral scientist. An interim letter with preliminary results was sent in January 2012.

At the time of our site visit, the steel mill produced electrical and stainless steel coils 24 hours a day, 7 days a week and employed approximately 1,200 hourly employees on three 8-hour shifts. Scrap metal was delivered by trucks. A crane operator loaded the scrap metal onto train cars that were driven to the melt shop and unloaded into one of the furnaces. The metal was melted down, poured into vats, and analyzed. If necessary, the composition was changed by adding ingredients. The molten metal was then cast into rectangular slabs that were loaded onto train cars and transported to the milling area. The slab was run through rollers to press the metal into a thin, long sheet and then rolled into a coil. The coils were taken to the finishing area, wrapped with metal ribbon, and shipped in trailer trucks.

All steel mill employees were required to wear a specific type of cut-resistant sleeve to prevent cuts and scratches common in this industry. No other types of sleeves were provided to employees. This policy had been implemented about 3 years before our evaluation. The union reported that, prior to this policy, employees wore other types of cut-resistant sleeves including a grey sleeve composed of mostly Kevlar®, and not all employees were required to wear them. The manufacturer of the current cut-resistant sleeves reported that the sleeves were made of a blended weave of para-aramid (Kevlar), cellulose, and E-glass fibers. New sleeves emitted very few fibers into the air under controlled use conditions [AM Health and Safety 2011]. However, employees were concerned that the sleeves could shed respirable fiberglass fibers, that this shedding could increase after repeated launderings, and that this exposure could cause skin irritation, respiratory irritation, or chronic respiratory disease. Some employees had safety concerns about wearing the sleeves, including the sleeve clips getting caught on machinery, and the sleeve fabric over the hand, when worn with gloves, interfering with grip and causing hand and wrist pain. After the employer received some employee complaints about skin discomfort from wearing these sleeves, a new policy was implemented that required employees to wear a long sleeve cotton shirt (100% cotton Indura flame resistant fabric by Westex Inc., Chicago, Illinois) underneath the cut-resistant sleeves. Despite this policy, employee concerns continued. Union representatives stated that the departments with the most employee complaints about the protective sleeves included the melt shop and melt shop maintenance, the hot mill and hot mill maintenance, shipping, and transportation. We focused our evaluation on these departments.

Methods

Our main objectives were to assess the potential of the cut-resistant sleeves to shed fiberglass fibers onto skin, clothing, and work surfaces, to evaluate whether employee reports of skin and respiratory symptoms could be related to fiberglass exposure, and, if fiberglass fibers were being shed, assess whether these fibers presented a short-term or long-term health hazard. We evaluated the size and morphology of collected fibers to assess the risk of potential skin and respiratory symptoms and illness. We also wanted to determine if wear and tear from repeated use or laundering could cause fiberglass fiber breakage that could compromise the cut resistance of the sleeves.

Qualitative Surface and Skin Fiber Sampling

There are no standard methods for surface sampling of fiberglass fibers, so we adapted published methods for other substances for our evaluation. Tape sampling was selected because gelatin tape sampling has been used to sample man-made fibers in an office building [Salonen et al. 2009], and to study mold on surfaces [Urzì and De Leo 2001; Krause et al. 2006]. Tape has been shown to be an easy and fast method to sample surfaces [Urzì and De Leo 2001]. One study reported that vacuum sampling was comparable to wipe sampling for asbestos; however, vacuum sampling was more efficient on the rough surfaces tested [Kominsky and Millette 2010]. Therefore, we also used vacuum sampling.

On October 25–26, 2011, we collected fiber samples using either tape or vacuum sampling from surfaces suspected of potentially having fibers from the cut-resistant sleeves. This included work surfaces, clothing, and skin. Samples were collected from different locations in the steel mill to determine if fibers were being shed in different areas. A new pair of nitrile gloves was used when collecting each sample to avoid cross contamination. Two field blank samples for each method were collected by exposing the media briefly to ambient air. Appendix A describes the tape and vacuum sampling methods. We did not perform air sampling for fibers because a steel mill contractor documented that the new cut-resistant sleeves emitted very few fibers (0.07 to 0.22 fibers per cubic centimeter of air) under controlled use conditions [AM Health and Safety 2011].

Bulk Sampling

Three new and two laundered cut-resistant sleeves were collected and sent to the laboratory for analysis. Of the three new sleeves, two were provided during our site visit, and the third sleeve was provided by union representatives after our site visit to determine potential variations due to different manufacturing batches. Both laundered sleeves were collected from the silicon building in the steel mill.

Fibers from the sleeves were compared with other fibers found in the steel mill. Other sources of fibers identified in the facility included yellow insulation used in roofs and pipelines (glass wool) and white fibrous material (Kaowool), which is used for thermal insulation of ovens and other industrial equipment, expansion relief, or packing behind brickwork in furnaces.

Qualitative Fiber Analysis

Surface and bulk samples were analyzed by stereomicroscope and polarized light microscopy for identification of fiberglass, Kevlar, cellulose, or other fibrous components of the sleeves, and for fiber morphology and size (Appendix A). Laboratory data provided percentages of each of the fiber types. Because the analysis was qualitative, we cannot calculate surface loading (number of fibers per area sampled).

Manufacturer's Analysis of Cut-resistant Properties

The manufacturer of the cut-resistant sleeves analyzed laundered sleeves for cut resistance properties to see if the steel mill's laundering procedure or number of launderings had affected the sleeve's intended cut-resistant properties. The manufacturer recommends washing the sleeves with commercial laundry soap or detergent in warm water not to exceed 140°F, rinsing in 160°F water, rinsing again in cold water, and tumbling dry in temperatures not to exceed 180°F. No chlorine bleach or dry cleaning solutions should be used. When laundered according to these instructions, the manufacturer has determined that the cut-resistant properties are preserved within 10 laundry cycles. We collected an additional nine laundered sleeves from different areas in the mill (silicon, shipping, hot mill maintenance, transportation, and melt shop) for this analysis. The manufacturer performed cut resistance testing (ASTM F1790-97 method) and abrasion resistance testing (ASTM D3389-05 method) [ASTM 1997, 2005].

Medical Interviews

We confidentially interviewed employees from the melt shop and melt shop maintenance, the hot mill and hot mill maintenance, shipping, and transportation departments. Interviewed employees were selected from a company roster and a list provided by the union. Most of the employees we interviewed worked on the day shift (7 a.m. to 3 p.m.) because this shift had the largest number of employees. We also interviewed some evening shift employees from the shipping department. We selected the employees off the roster and attempted to speak to everyone we selected. Some employees declined to be interviewed based on their availability. We asked about their work history, work exposures, personal protective equipment use, if they had concerns about wearing the cut-resistant sleeves, and if they had any health problems they thought were related to wearing the sleeves.

Health and Safety Concerns

Interviewed employees were also asked to respond to the following questions: (1) "How much are you concerned about your health?" (2) "How stressful is your job?" and (3) "How much confidence or trust do you have in management to look out for your well-being?" Employees were instructed to use a scale from 1 to 10, where 1 indicated "very little," and 10 indicated "very much." A NIOSH behavioral scientist who specializes in job stress and work organization issues evaluated the employees' responses.

Review of Medical Records and Occupational Safety and Health Administration 300 Injury and Illness Logs

We reviewed medical records of employees who had seen a medical care provider for an illness or injury they felt was related to work. We also reviewed the steel mill's Occupational

Safety and Health Administration (OSHA) 300 Injury and Illness Logs and company first aid logs for years 2008 to 2011.

Review of Ergonomic Concerns

We asked a NIOSH ergonomist to review photos and information on job tasks performed by masonry employees and personal protective equipment they wore, including gloves. We wanted to better understand how the use of cut-resistant sleeves in conjunction with heavy protective gloves may affect grip strength.

Results

Observations

All employees were required to wear the cut-resistant sleeves; these were the only type available to employees at the time of our evaluation. Employees obtained new sleeves from dispenser machines located in only a few places throughout the facility (Figure 1). New sleeves were also available without a dispenser in other areas of the steel mill. Sleeves were also reused after being laundered. Employees placed soiled sleeves in designated bins after use (Figure 2), and the soiled sleeves were sent to a contracted laundry service. A company manager provided us with the washing and drying procedures used by this laundry service when laundering the cut-resistant sleeves. These instructions were identical to the manufacturer's recommendations. Laundered sleeves were available in various locations of the steel mill (Figure 3). From our observations and from talking to the employer and to employees, we learned that sleeves were laundered without tracking the number of cleaning cycles and that some employees laundered their sleeves at home. Some of these laundered sleeves had visible holes and stains, suggesting that the sleeves were not adequately inspected and taken out of service. We observed that some employee locker rooms did not provide easy employee access to either new or laundered sleeves. The employer said that they were planning to increase the number of dispensers throughout the steel mill and keep track of the number of sleeves an employee used.

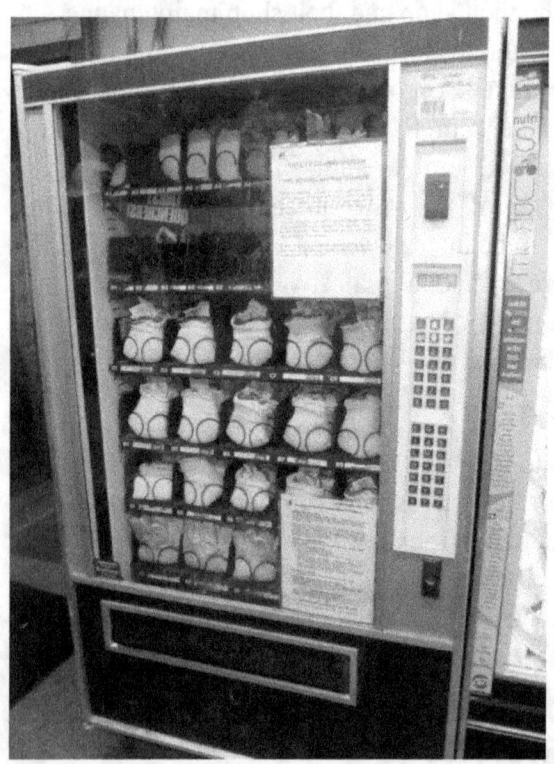

Figure 1. Dispenser for new gloves and cut-resistant sleeves.

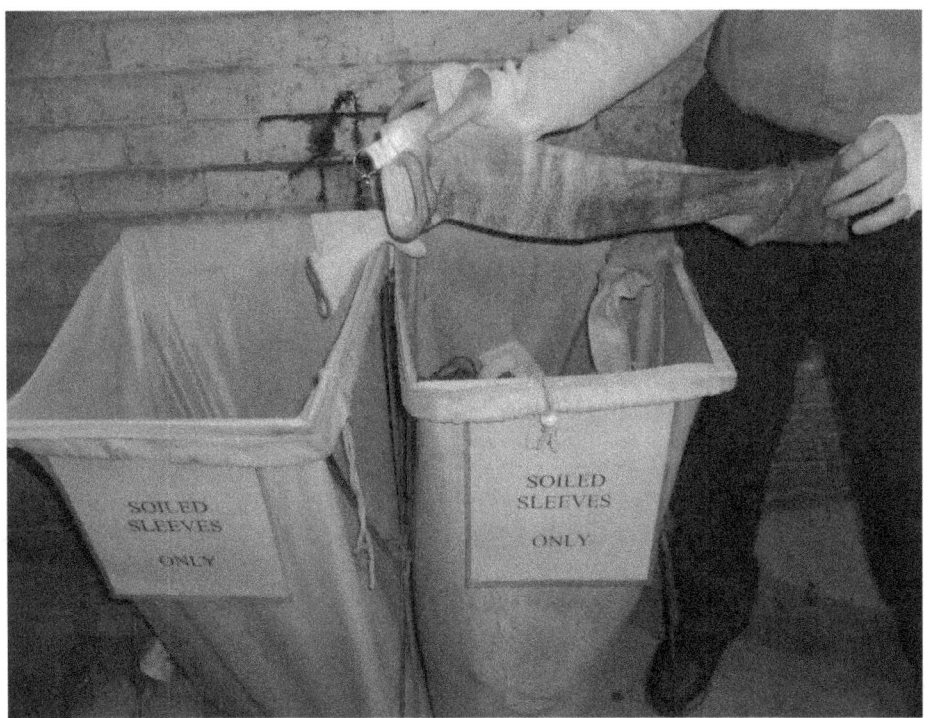

Figure 2. Bins where soiled cut-resistant sleeves were collected near the production area.

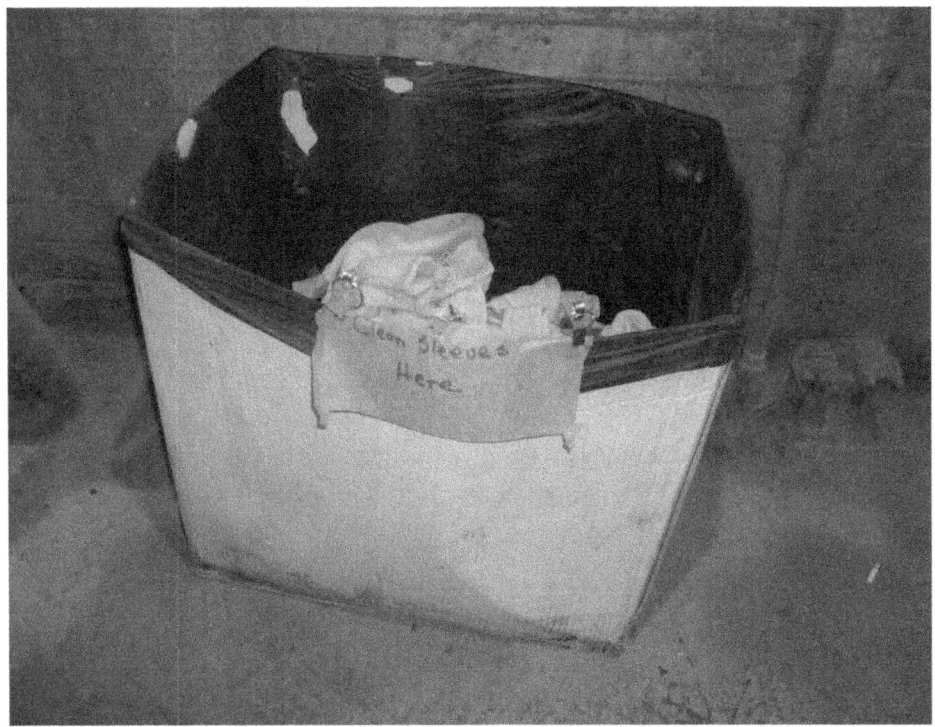

Figure 3. Box where laundered sleeves were stored near the production area.

Qualitative Surface and Skin Fiber Sampling

We collected 4 surface, 33 clothing, and 6 skin samples. Surface samples included those surfaces where sleeves were stored, such as plastic or cloth bags. Clothing surfaces included cut-resistant sleeves or shirts worn under the sleeves. Of the 15 employees we included in this sampling, 60% reported using new (unlaundered) sleeves, and 40% reported using laundered sleeves. Those employees who used new sleeves reported using them an average of 6 days, while those who used laundered sleeves reported using them an average of 7 days before replacing them. Skin surface samples included hands and forearms of sleeve users.

Table B1 (Appendix B) presents the fiber results from all surface samples collected using the tape method (cut-resistant sleeves, clothing, and skin) and Table B2 (Appendix B) presents results from all surface samples collected using the vacuum method (cut-resistant sleeves, clothing, and skin). Tape samples contained fiberglass, Kevlar, and/or cellulose fibers. Vacuum samples contained fiberglass and/or cellulose fibers. Where present, the Kevlar fibers averaged 20 μm in width, and the fiberglass fibers averaged 10 μm in width. Both the Kevlar and fiberglass fibers had variable lengths. Fiber size and shape were similar for both new and laundered sleeve samples. None of the Kevlar, fiberglass, or cellulose fibers seen in these surface samples had sharp edges. (No material was observed on the media blanks and field blanks for vacuum samples. The tape field blanks contained fiberglass and cellulose fibers, but Kevlar fibers were not observed. Neither the vacuum nor tape media blanks had fibers.)

Bulk Analysis

Photomicrographs of the different bulk samples and summary results and photomicrographs of the fiber analysis for the new and laundered cut-resistant sleeves are presented in Appendix C, Figures C1–C10. Photomicrographs display the different parts of the sleeves from the outside and the inside of the sleeve. Only one sample of each of the sleeves is presented for conciseness. Table B3 (Appendix B) presents the bulk analysis summary results for the fiber composition of the new and laundered sleeves.

Regardless of whether the cut-resistant sleeve was new or laundered, some of the Kevlar and fiberglass bundles in the sleeves were frayed and broken in many areas (Figures C3–C8).

Other sources of fiber in the steel mill were yellow insulation composed of 100% glass wool and white fibrous material composed of 99% Kaowool and 1% cellulose fiber. Photomicrographs of the fiber analysis for the yellow and white insulation are included in Figures C11–C14 (Appendix C). Glass wool and Kaowool fibers were not found in any of the sleeve or surface samples.

Manufacturer's Analysis of Cut-resistant Properties

The manufacturer of the cut-resistant sleeves determined that the nine samples of laundered sleeves maintained their cut and abrasion resistant properties; however, the number of laundry cycles they had been through was unknown. The manufacturer reported that many of the sleeves were not adequately cleaned and the washing procedures could be improved for cleanliness and appearance.

Medical Interviews

We interviewed 54 of 92 available employees from the areas of concern during our site visit: 16 of 29 hot mill employees (including hot mill operators and hot mill maintenance employees), 22 of 41 melt shop employees (including melt shop operators and helpers, melt shop maintenance employees, and masonry employees), 9 of 9 transportation employees, and 7 of 13 shipping department employees. The average age of these employees was 50 years (range: 37 to 62 years), and the average number of years worked at the steel mill was 20 years (range: < 1 year to 38 years).

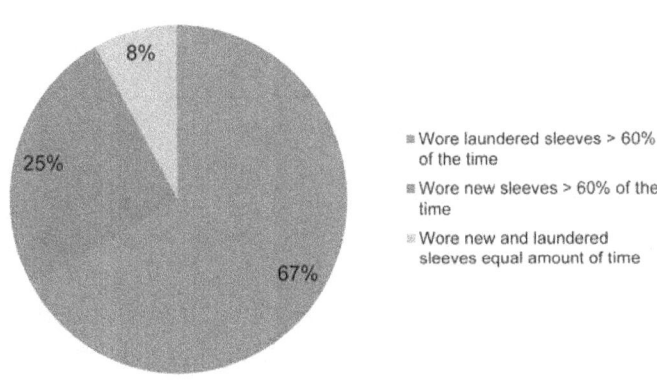

Figure 4. New vs. laundered sleeve use among interviewed employees.

We asked employees about the use of new versus laundered sleeves (Figure 4). We asked how many shifts they wore a pair of sleeves before getting another pair (Figure 5). Forty-eight employees responded. Most employees wore laundered sleeves and most employees wore their sleeves more than one day. Nine employees reported that they took sleeves home to launder.

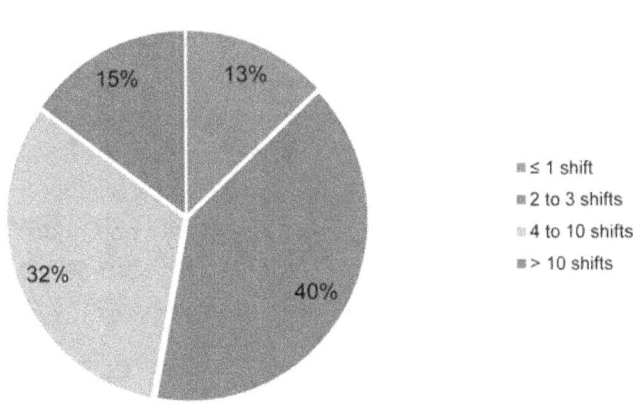

Figure 5. Number of shifts employees wore a pair of sleeves before getting another pair.

When asked the question, "Do you have any health problems you think are related to work at [the steel mill]," 14 employees responded "Yes" and 14 employees responded "Unsure." Employees who reported having any type of work-related health problem, or who were unsure if the health problem was related to work, were asked about their symptoms during the month prior to our visit (Table 1). Those who answered "No" were considered to not have any symptoms. Headache and nose and eye irritation were the most commonly reported symptoms among these employees, and most reported that these symptoms improved away from work.

Table 1. Interviewed employees reporting symptoms in the month prior to our visit (N=54)

Symptoms	Employees reporting symptom No. (%)	Employees reporting symptom improves away from work No.(%)
Headache	13 (24)	10 of 13 (76)
Nasal irritation	12 (22)	11 of 12 (92)
Eye irritation	10 (19)	8 of 10 (80)
Throat irritation	6 (11)	4 of 6 (67)
Cough	6 (11)	3 of 6 (50)
Shortness of breath	4 (7)	2 of 4 (50)
Wheeze	3 (6)	1 of 3 (33)
Chest tightness	2 (4)	1 of 2 (50)

We asked employees if they had any additional concerns about the use of the cut-resistant sleeves. Most of the interviewed employees were concerned about the sleeves being uncomfortably hot and causing more sweating. Others had safety concerns, reporting that sleeves would catch on things. One fifth of interviewed employees reported that their gloves didn't fit well when using the sleeves and some (particularly among the masonry employees) felt that their grip was compromised, causing hand pain and numbness. Skin itch without rash due to the sleeves was reported by four employees. Hygiene was also a concern; employees reported that it was difficult to wash their hands properly and that the sleeves got dirty but they were required to wear them between the location where they washed their hands and the lunchroom. Several also felt that the sleeves were not laundered properly. Others were concerned that breathing in fiberglass fibers from the sleeves could be harmful to their lungs over time.

Masonry employees reported that there was a recent change in the type of glove provided to them. They reported the newer gloves were bulkier and had a flannel covering that was slippery, which led to poor grip and difficulty feeling the brick. These employees reported the use of the sleeves and gloves together resulted in a tight feeling around the hands that restricted movement, and some employees reported hand numbness, and hand, wrist, and outer elbow pain. They also reported there had been a prior exception to the mandatory sleeve policy for masonry employees stating that the cut-resistant sleeves were not required to be worn during handling, laying, cutting, or hammering bricks. Reportedly, this policy was revoked.

Health and Safety Concerns

The results of employee responses to three questions concerning health and safety concerns and stress at work are presented in Table 2.

With respect to health concerns, 46 (87%) employees gave a rating of 8 or more, indicating a great deal of concern for one's health. Job stress was also rated high, with 36 (68%) employees indicating a rating of 8 or greater. Thirty-six (68%) employees rated their trust in the employer to care for their well-being as 3 or less.

Table 2. Employee health concerns, perceptions of job stress, and trust in management (N=53)

Question	Average response	Most frequent response	Response range*
How much are you concerned about your health?	9.2	10	3–10
How stressful is your job?	7.7	10	1–10
How much confidence or trust do you have in management to look out for your well-being?	2.9	1	1–10

*Response scale was 1 to 10; 1 indicated "very little," and 10 indicated "very much."

Interviewed employees expressed additional concerns about safety climate. Employees reported frequent punishment (e.g., being "written up," docked hours, or fired) for mistakes, errors in procedures (e.g., personal protective equipment use), and injuries. Some employees believed that frequent disciplinary action was due to supervisors being required to fulfill a "disciplinary quota." This was brought up in the closing meeting and managers believed that this perception was due to routine safety checks performed by supervisors where the result was not necessarily disciplinary action.

Several employees expressed feelings that the employer did not have the individual employees' well-being in mind, but were instead focused on the company's interests (e.g., production and potential liability) before concerns for the employees' health and safety. Some employees also felt that the employer's efforts to control personal protective equipment use (particularly the cut-resistant sleeves, which were perceived as unnecessary in some positions/roles) overshadowed a variety of other health and safety issues. Further, employees felt that the safety management team did not address health and safety concerns raised by employees.

Review of Medical Records

Medical records for six employees were reviewed. There were no findings of health problems related to the cut-resistant sleeves.

Review of Injury and Illness Logs

The type and number of entries from the recordable (OSHA) and non-recordable injury and illness logs are shown in Table B4 (Appendix B). The most common entries in both logs were lacerations, abrasions, punctures, and contusions. During 2008, the required use of cut-resistant sleeves was introduced. The total number of lacerations, abrasions, punctures, and contusions per year went from seven in 2008 to three in 2009, but back up to six in 2010 and five in 2011.

Comparing Non-Fatal Injury and Illness Rates Between the Pennsylvania Steel Mill and the U.S. Iron and Steel Mills Manufacturing Industry

We used data from the OSHA Logs to calculate and compare incidence rates of nonfatal injury and illness between this mill and the U.S. iron and steel mill manufacturing industry as a whole (NAICS Code 331111) [BLS 2010]. The incidence rates are for nonfatal injuries and illnesses per 100 full-time employees for each year (Table 3). These rates can be useful for determining problem areas and progress in preventing work-related injuries and illnesses and showing comparisons across similar industries. These rates are calculated using the following formula:

Incidence rate = number of injuries and illnesses × 200,000 / employee hours worked

The 200,000 hours in the formula represents the equivalent of 100 employees working 40 hours a week, 50 weeks a year. We estimated the number of the steel mill's employees for 2010 to be 1,160 (on the basis of 1,162 hourly workers employed during our site visit in 2011). The steel mill had 8 recordable cases out of approximately 1,160 employees in 2010, which is equivalent to 0.7 recordable cases per 100 employees. We used the number of work hours per week as 40 hours a week, the standard formula number of 200,000 hours, to allow comparison to other plants with the same NAICS code throughout the United States.

Table 3. Comparison of nonfatal injury and illness incidence rates (for total recordable cases in the steel mill and all U.S. iron and steel mills) per 100 full-time employees for 2010

	Steel mill*	All U.S. iron and steel mills
Total recordable cases	0.7	3.6
Cases involving days away from work	0.3	0.8
Cases involving days of job transfer or restriction	0.2	1.0
Cases involving days away from work, job restriction, or transfer	0.5	1.8

*Assuming hourly workers = 1,160; working 40 hours a week, 50 weeks per year

Table B5 (Appendix B) presents data for the industry on the rates of workplace injuries and illnesses per 100 full-time workers in primary metal manufacturing. An injury or illness is considered to be work-related if an event or exposure in the work environment either caused or contributed to the resulting condition or significantly aggravated a pre-existing condition.

When we compare the industry rates to the steel mill rates, the industry's rates are tenfold higher for total recordable cases. Figure 6 compares the total OSHA recordable cases and cases with "days away from work, restricted work activity, or job transfer" (DART) between the steel mill and U.S. industry for years 2008-2010. Trends in the steel mill's injury and illness rates could indicate an actual lower number of recordable events as compared to the industry or may be due to consistent underreporting or lack of documentation.

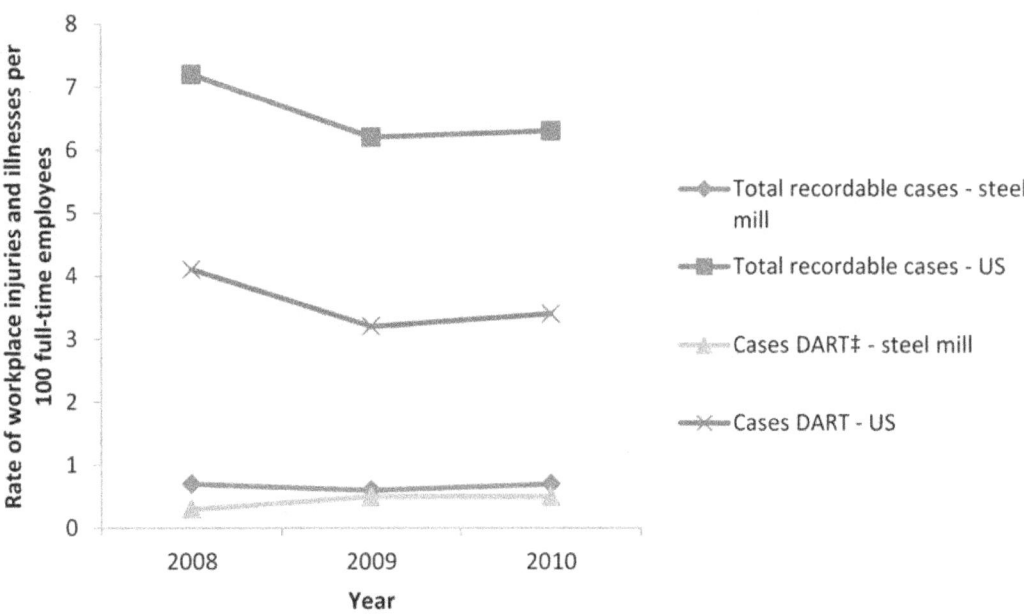

Figure 6. Comparing rates of workplace injuries and illnesses per 100 full-time workers between the steel mill* and U.S. iron and steel mills† (NAICS 331111), years 2008–2010.

*On the basis of 1,160 steel mill employees per year at this facility
†From Bureau of Labor Statistics (BLS) website:
http://www.bls.gov/iag/tgs/iag331.htm#fatalities_injuries_and_illnesses
‡Cases with days away from work, restricted work activity, or job transfer

Review of Ergonomic Concerns

Our ergonomist reviewed photos of masonry employees performing tasks wearing the required personal protective equipment. The photos showed masonry employees wearing cut-resistant sleeves under work gloves and lifting, holding, stacking, and positioning large oven bricks that the union reported to weigh between 40 and 70 pounds.

Discussion

On the basis of requestor concerns, our main goal for this HHE was to determine if the cut-resistant sleeves were shedding fiberglass fibers and, if so, whether these fibers presented a short-term or long-term health hazard. We found that fiberglass fibers were shed from both new and laundered sleeves. Fiberglass, Kevlar, and cellulose fibers were found on work surfaces, on shirt sleeves under the protective sleeves, and on employee's skin.

We analyzed the size and other characteristics of these fibers to determine if they posed a health hazard. Fibers found on surfaces, shirt sleeves, and skin were of the same material and width as those from the sleeves. Kevlar fibers had an average width of 20 μm, and fiberglass had an average width of 10 μm. The fibers had variable lengths. We did not find glass wool or Kaowool fibers in our samples, which are the fibers found in insulation throughout the steel mill. Furthermore, other sources of fiber in the steel mill did not seem to contribute to the fibers found in the surfaces tested.

The fiberglass, Kevlar, and cellulose fibers found in the samples are not classified as human carcinogens [ACGIH 2011; NTP 2011]. On the basis of a review of the scientific literature, fibers with a width larger than 3 μm deposit in the upper airways and are not considered respirable (able to penetrate deep into the lungs) [ATSDR 2002; ACGIH 2011]. In addition, the large size of the fiberglass and Kevlar fibers shed from the sleeves makes the fibers unlikely to remain airborne for long periods of time; therefore, we do not expect the fiberglass or Kevlar fibers found on work surfaces, cut-resistant sleeves, or skin to pose an inhalation hazard or cause any long-term respiratory effects [ATSDR 2002; ACGIH 2011].

No consistent evidence of an increased risk of respiratory disease or death due to glass fiber exposure has been found among studies of fiberglass manufacturing workers (with high levels of exposure) in Europe or North America [Hesterberg and Hart 2001]. However, fiberglass fibers may cause reversible upper airway irritation [Hesterberg and Hart 2001] and reversible skin irritation in some individuals [Heisel and Hunt 1968; Possick et al. 1970; Hsieh et al. 2001]. Thus, fiberglass exposure could explain reports of eye, nose, throat, and skin irritation from some interviewed employees at the steel mill; however, these symptoms could also be caused or exacerbated by other factors such as dust and smoke exposure.

Employee interviews revealed several additional concerns about the use of the cut-resistant sleeves, including safety, hygiene, availability, cleanliness, steam burns, and possible musculoskeletal disorders from wearing the sleeves during certain job tasks. The cleanliness concerns agreed with our field observations and those of the manufacturer when analyzing the sleeves for cut resistance. Also, some employees were taking their sleeves home to be laundered. This could affect the protective properties if sleeves are not laundered per the manufacturer's instructions and could potentially contaminate the home with fibers that could be irritating to family members.

Masonry employees reported the most hand and wrist pain and numbness from wearing the sleeves under their heavy work gloves. Ergonomic studies of gloves have shown that thick gloves result in increased hand fatigue, reduced gripping power, and decreased tactile sensitivity. Because the sleeve material also covers the hand up to the fingers, the sleeve under the glove can compound the problems of wearing a thick glove. Glove use decreases hand grip and forearm strength; the thicker the glove, the weaker the grip strength [Wimer et al. 2010]. Glove use also increases muscle activity, wrist posture, and discomfort. The longer the duration of work tasks using gloves, the greater effect the gloves have on hand performance capabilities. In general, gloves lessen skin sensation and increase grip force [Dianat et al. 2012]. Smooth gloves tend to increase grip forces to prevent slippage [Wimer et al. 2010; Dianat et al. 2012]. Textured gloves reduce the forces needed for grasping [Kopka et al. 2005; Chang and Shih 2007; Laroche et al. 2007]. Additionally, the masonry workers occasionally exceeded the NIOSH recommended weight limit of 51 pounds [Waters et al. 1994], which could increase their risk of back pain, in addition to the risk of hand and wrist pain.

In general, the type of sleeve that should be worn is dictated by the job tasks of the employee. For example, it is possible that a shipping employee could wear a sleeve with different properties than a sleeve a melt shop employee would wear. In addition, the same type of sleeve may come in different styles so that it covers the arm and wrist, but not the hand, or covers the hand entirely, or covers the back of the hand but not the palm. These alternatives might be available to employees who have problems wearing the sleeves.

Interviews with employees revealed that a primary contributing factor to job stress was what they considered to be a top-down management system that was perceived as punitive in nature. This perception of the management style may also explain why employees reported low trust in management. Our review of OSHA Logs showed rates of injury and illness at this steel mill to be one tenth the rate of other steel mill manufacturing plants in the United States. This may show a better than average safety record in this specific facility; however, it may reflect underreporting of injuries and illnesses because of employees' fear of retaliation from management. Comments made by employees during the interviews support the possibility of underreporting of injuries and illnesses.

Conclusions

We found that the cut-resistant sleeves shed fiberglass fibers, but the size and other characteristics of the shed fiberglass fibers make them unlikely to cause any long-term health effects. However, the fibers may cause or contribute to employee reports of skin, eye, nose, and throat irritation. Employees whose job tasks require hand, wrist, and finger strength, such as masonry work, may have more problems when wearing protective sleeves that cover the hand and heavy gloves. This combination could add to forces required to grip heavy objects and could have led to or aggravated the symptoms of hand and wrist pain and numbness reported by masonry employees. It could also lead to or aggravate other work-related musculoskeletal disorders. Additionally, a lack of trust in management was widespread among employees, and many felt that the employer did not address health and safety concerns raised by employees.

Recommendations

On the basis of our findings, we recommend the actions listed below. We encourage the steel mill to use a labor-management health and safety committee or working group to discuss the recommendations and develop an action plan. Those involved in the work can best set priorities and assess the feasibility of our recommendations for the specific situation at the steel mill.

Our recommendations are based on an approach known as the hierarchy of controls. This approach groups actions by their likely effectiveness in reducing or removing hazards. In most cases, the preferred approach is to eliminate hazardous materials or processes and install engineering controls to reduce exposure or shield employees. Until such controls are in place, or if they are not effective or feasible, administrative measures and personal protective equipment may be needed.

Elimination and Substitution

Eliminating or substituting hazardous processes or materials reduces hazards and protects employees more effectively than other approaches. Prevention through design, considering elimination or substitution when designing or developing a project, reduces the need for additional controls in the future.

1. Provide employees who have health or safety concerns about the cut-resistant sleeves with alternative sleeves that have appropriate levels of protection for their job tasks.

2. Provide masonry employees with alternative gloves that have appropriate protection for their job tasks, preferably thinner, more durable gloves with better grip and longer cuffs. Consider testing gloves for dexterity and grip based on the National Fire Protection Association (NFPA) Glove Hand Function and Grip Tests which would be helpful in determining the most appropriate gloves for masonry job tasks [NFPA 2006]. A description of these test methods is given in Chapter 8 of the NFPA Standard

Engineering Controls

Engineering controls reduce exposures to employees by removing the hazard from the process or placing a barrier between the hazard and the employee. Engineering controls are very effective at protecting employees without placing primary responsibility of implementation on the employee.

1. Provide an adjustable power lift assist device and place brick pallets on the lift so the bricks are around waist height. This will minimize bending.

Administrative Controls

The term administrative controls refer to employer-dictated work practices and policies to reduce or prevent hazardous exposures. Their effectiveness depends on employer commitment and employee acceptance. Regular monitoring and reinforcement are necessary to ensure that policies and procedures are followed consistently.

1. Reconsider the plant-wide policy on wearing the cut-resistant sleeves. Define the areas where most lacerations occur, and determine if the other areas need the sleeve requirement. Include input from employees.

2. Develop a committee with union and employer representation to discuss personal protective equipment issues and determine what type of alternatives could be provided. This committee can work to identify a solution for the masonry employees to combine the use of appropriately protective gloves and sleeves that will reduce or prevent hand, wrist, and arm pain and numbness.

3. Provide new and laundered cut-resistant sleeves in more easily accessible locations throughout the steel mill, including employee locker rooms.

4. Prohibit employees from taking the cut-resistant sleeves home for laundering.

5. Keep track of the number of laundry cycles for the sleeves and follow manufacturer's guidelines on replacement.

6. Train employees in proper care, maintenance, useful life, and disposal of sleeves. Employees should inspect sleeves before wearing to make sure they are not torn or damaged and should notify their supervisor of the need to replace sleeves.

7. Audit laundered sleeves regularly to ensure they are being cleaned appropriately. The manufacturer notes that when laundering heavily soiled sleeves, an additional wash and rinse cycle may be needed, and adding several pieces of heavy canvas in the second wash cycle helps loosen and remove the deep dirt.

8. Continue encouraging the use of long sleeve shirts under the cut-resistant sleeves to minimize direct contact of the sleeve material with the skin. Shirts should be made from flame-resistant cotton, wool, or Nomex®. Fabrics containing polyester, nylon, and other materials with relatively low melting points should be avoided because these increase the injury in a burn or heat situation.

9. Encourage employees, especially those with skin irritation, to shower before leaving the work environment [NIOSH 1997].

10. Consider providing uniforms and/or coveralls with laundry service to steel mill production employees to prevent workplace contaminants from contacting skin and street clothing. Ensure that a laundering procedure is used that will remove fibers. Keep in mind that flame-resistant cotton uses a treatment which will be removed over time with launderings, especially when laundered with high temperatures and aggressive chemicals.

11. Provide hand washing facilities in break areas to allow employees to clean their hands and arms before eating, drinking, or smoking.

12. Train employees on the proper use of the cut resistant sleeves. Include information on the protective characteristics of the sleeves, inspection of sleeves, restrictions on taking them home, health and safety practices, and good personal hygiene practices.

13. Encourage masonry employees to avoid rushing, get help when needed, avoid twisting when performing a lift, and keep the load close to their body [Waters et al. 1994].

14. Improve communication between the employer and employees regarding responses to employee safety and health concerns. A management or union representative of the safety management team should communicate directly with employees who report health and safety concerns to let the employees know that their input has been received and what will be done to address the concern. If nothing will be done to address the concern, this should also be communicated and the rationale given to provide closure.

15. Develop a safety climate that encourages safe behaviors and the reporting of safety-related issues. A consultant may be useful in developing a positive safety climate. The Society for Industrial and Organizational Psychology maintains a consultant locator at http://www.siop.org/consultantlocator/search.aspx. The American Society of Safety Engineers also maintains directories of qualified consultants at http://www.asse.org/practicespecialties/consultants/.

Appendix A: Methods

Qualitative Surface and Skin Fiber Sampling

Tape sampling

Stick-to-it lift tape (part number 225-9809, SKC Inc., Eighty Four, Pennsylvania) was used following manufacturer instructions [SKC 2011]. The protective liner of the slide was peeled off to expose the adhesive. Then the slide was placed sticky side down on the surface to be sampled while we gently pressed down to ensure contact (Figure A1). The slide was carefully removed, placed back in the slide mailer, and labeled. Figure A2 shows a tape being used to sample on an employee's uniform sleeve after he had removed the cut-resistant sleeves.

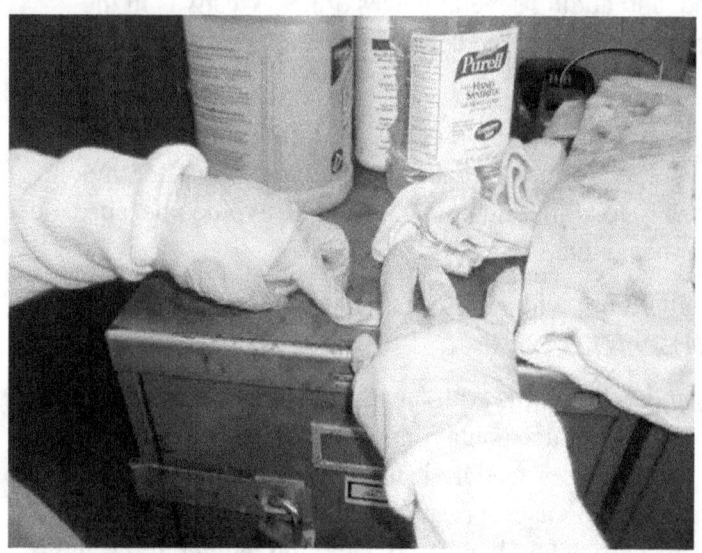

Figure A1. Tape sampling of a surface where cut-resistant sleeves were stored.

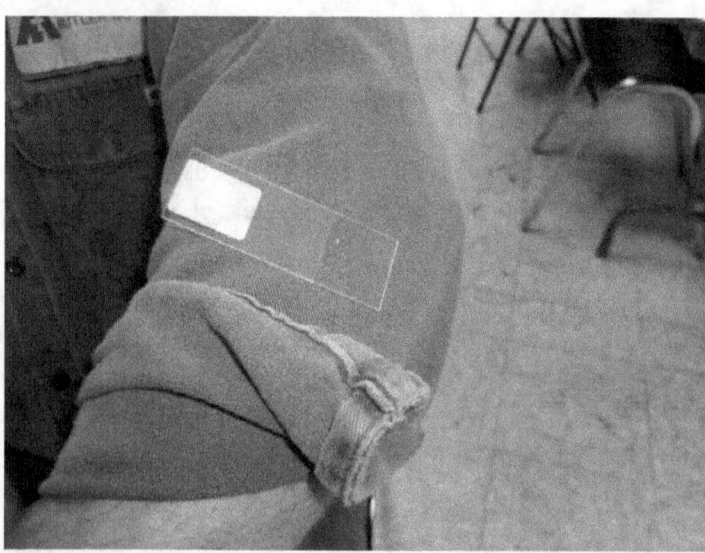

Figure A2. Tape sampling on employee's uniform sleeves after removing the cut-resistant sleeve.

Vacuum Sampling

Polycarbonate filters (37 millimeter, 0.8 micrometer [μm], SKC Inc., Eighty Four, Pennsylvania) were used with cellulose back-up pads inside conductive three-piece cassettes. Air was drawn through the cassette at 15 liters per minute by an SKC QuickTake 30 pump. Sampling was similar to that described by NIOSH Method 7400 for asbestos and other fibers [NIOSH 2013]. However, an open cassette instead of a closed cassette with a nozzle was used to avoid any losses because of static typical of fiberglass.

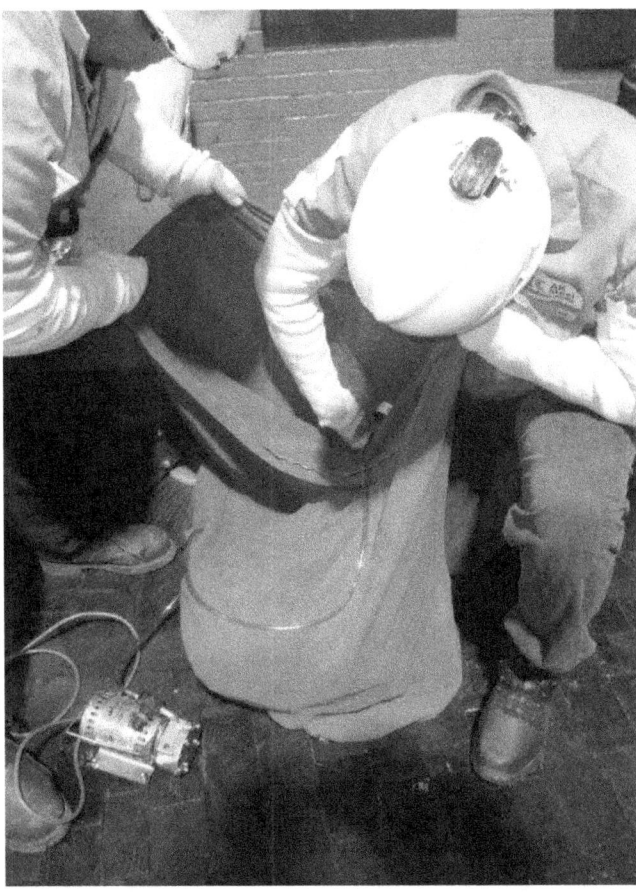

Figure A3. Vacuum sampling of the surface of a bag that stored new cut-resistant sleeves.

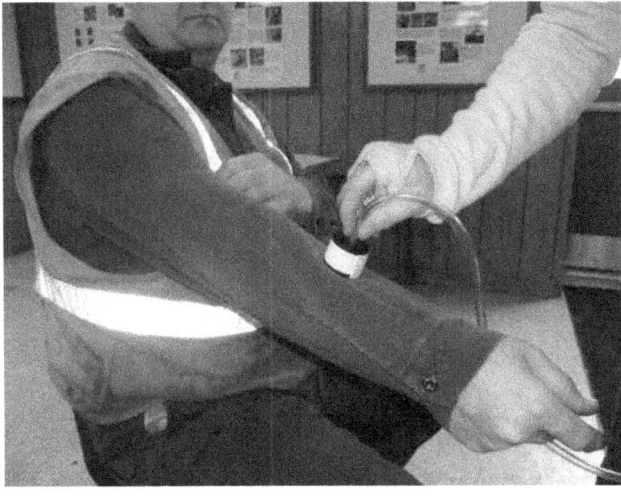

Figure A4. Vacuum sampling on an employee's uniform sleeve after removing the cut-resistant sleeve.

A surface was selected, and 100-square-centimeter disposable cardboard templates were used when possible for consistency. When a guide was not possible because of an irregular shape, vacuuming for 1 minute (for an approximate volume of 15 liters of air) was performed. The cassette was placed at an angle with the surface to avoid a pump fault. The cassette was used in an overlapping "S" pattern to vacuum the entire surface with horizontal strokes. The same area was vacuumed again using vertical S-strokes and diagonal S-strokes. Figures A3 and A4 show vacuum sampling of different surfaces.

Qualitative Fiber Analysis

Samples were analyzed by stereomicroscope and polarized light microscopy for identification of any fiberglass, Kevlar, and cellulose fibers (components of the cut-resistant sleeves), as well as for particle morphology and size [McCrone 1980; EPA 1982, 1993; Bureau Veritas North America 2000]. Samples were first examined by stereomicroscope to determine if any material was present and at what percent. The material of all filter samples was picked off the filter with forceps and mounted on glass slides in oil. For tape samples, only when the identification of the materials could not be resolved, the material was picked out of the tape with forceps and mounted on glass slides in oil. The mounts were then examined by polarized light microscopy to identify fibers on the basis of unique optical properties. For the bulk samples, each sleeve was examined and analyzed by polarized light microscopy and stereomicroscope to determine fiber identification, morphology, and size. A representative portion of the bulk sample was examined by polarized light microscopy to identify fibers on the basis of unique optical properties.

For all vacuum, tape, and bulk samples, birefringence, sign of elongation, dispersion staining, and other techniques aided the analyst in establishing the properties of the particle. Shape and color also helped to identify a particle. More than 100 standards on file were used as reference materials. Because no sample contained large amounts of particulate less than 5 μm in width, scanning electron microscope-energy dispersive spectroscopy was not done.

Appendix B: Tables

Table B1. Tape surface sampling fiber analysis results*

Sample location	Steel mill location	Percent fiber composition					
		Fiberglass	Kevlar	Cellulose	Synthetic	Hair	Others†
New sleeve	Hot mill	50	45	5	ND‡	ND	ND
	Hot mill	15	35	50	ND	ND	ND
	Melt shop	50	20	10	ND	ND	20
	Melt shop	35	45	10	ND	ND	10
	Shipping	35	35	30	ND	ND	ND
	Shipping	5	15	80	ND	ND	ND
Laundered sleeve	Hot mill	40	60	ND	ND	ND	ND
	Melt shop	35	30	35	ND	ND	ND
	Melt shop	35	40	25	ND	ND	ND
	Melt shop	45	50	5	ND	ND	ND
	Melt shop	40	55	5	ND	ND	ND
	Shipping	90	10	ND	ND	ND	ND
Shirt	Hot mill	2	43	55	ND	ND	ND
	Hot mill	2	45	53	ND	ND	ND
	Hot mill	10	45	45	ND	ND	ND
	Melt shop	20	40	40	ND	ND	ND
	Melt shop	2	49	49	ND	ND	ND
	Melt shop	10	ND	75	15	ND	ND
	Melt shop	5	35	60	ND	ND	ND
	Melt shop	5	2	88	5	ND	ND
	Shipping	3	95	2	ND	ND	ND
	Shipping	5	50	45	ND	ND	ND
	Shipping	2	ND	18	80	ND	ND
File cabinet where laundered sleeves stored	Hot Mill	2	ND	3	ND	ND	95
Plastic bag where laundered sleeves stored	Silicon	25	ND	75	ND	ND	ND
Back of hand	Melt shop	ND	ND	5	ND	ND	95
	Melt shop	ND	ND	2	ND	ND	98
Forearm	Melt shop	1	ND	10	ND	2	87
	Melt shop	5	ND	10	10	ND	75
	Shipping	ND	1	ND	ND	ND	99
	Shipping	1	ND	ND	1	ND	98
Missing data	Transportation	3	40	35	1	ND	21
	Transportation	45	45	10	ND	ND	ND

*Field blanks had 20%–25% fiberglass and 75%–80% cellulose.
†Other types of fibers include paint, opaque material, and plastic.
‡None detected

Table B2. Vacuum filter surface sampling fiber analysis results*

Sample location	Steel mill location	Percent fiber composition		
		Fiberglass	Cellulose	Opaque material
New sleeve	Hot mill	55	40	5
	Melt shop	30	30	40
Laundered sleeve	Hot mill	45	45	10
	Melt shop	20	50	30
	Melt shop	40	40	20
	Melt shop	10	40	50
	Shipping	40	50	10
Shirt	Hot mill	10	85	5
	Hot mill	10	10	80
	Melt shop	10	80	10
	Shipping	ND†	95	5
Bin where soiled sleeves were stored	Hot mill	5	50	45
Cloth bag holding new sleeves	Shipping	25	35	40
Missing data	Transportation	10	60	30
	Transportation	35	35	30

*Field blanks did not contain fibers

†None detected

Table B3. Summary fiber composition of new and laundered cut-resistant sleeves

Description	New sleeve	Laundered sleeve
Yellow hand cover	98%–100% 20 μm Kevlar	98%–99% 20 μm Kevlar
	0%–1% 10 μm fiberglass	0%–1% 10 μm fiberglass
	0%–1% cellulose	0%–1% cellulose
Yellow lining at thumb opening	99%–100% nylon	100% nylon
	0%–1% fiberglass	
Wrist seam	100% nylon	100% nylon
Yellow sleeve	50% 20 μm Kevlar	49%–50% 20 μm Kevlar
	49%–50% 10 μm fiberglass	49%–50% 10 μm fiberglass
	0%–1% cellulose fiber	0%–1% cellulose fiber
		0%–1% paint
Yellow seam inside upper arm opening	100% nylon	100% nylon
Yellow cuff inside upper arm	94%–95% 20 μm Kevlar	93% 20 μm Kevlar
	5% nylon	5% nylon
	0%–1% cellulose fiber	1% 10 μm fiberglass
		1% cellulose
White strap at upper arm opening	100% nylon	100% nylon

Table B4. Review of entries from OSHA Logs and the steel mill's non-recordable injury and illness logs, years 2008–2011

	2008		2009		2010		2011		Total
	OSHA	Non*	OSHA	Non*	OSHA	Non*	OSHA	Non*	
Laceration, abrasion, puncture, contusion	5	2	0	3	1	5	4	1	21
Eye injury	0	0	1	1	2	0	0	1	5
Fracture, amputation	3	0	2	1	3	0	1	0	10
Sprain, strain	0	0	2	3	1	2	0	1	9
Burn	0	0	1	1	0	0	0	2	4
Heat illness	0	0	0	0	1	0	1	0	2
Smoke inhalation	0	0	1	1	0	0	0	0	2
Skin disorder	0	0	0	1	0	1	0	0	2
Total	8	2	7	11	8	8	6	5	55

*Injuries and illnesses not required to be recorded on OSHA Log

Table B5. Comparing rates of workplace injuries and illnesses per 100 full-time workers between the steel mill* and U.S. iron and steel mills† (NAICS 331111), years 2008–2010

Data series	2008 mill	2008 U.S.	2009 mill	2009 U.S.	2010 mill	2010 U.S.
Total recordable cases	0.7	7.2	0.6	6.2	0.7	6.3
Cases involving days away from work	0.2	1.8	0.3	1.5	0.3	1.6
Cases involving days of job transfer or restriction	0.09	2.3	0.2	1.8	0.2	1.8
Cases involving days away from work, job restriction, or transfer	0.3	4.1	0.5	3.2	0.5	3.4

*On the basis of 1,160 steel mill employees per year at this facility

†From BLS website: http://www.bls.gov/iag/tgs/iag331.htm#fatalities_injuries_and_illnesses

Appendix C: Photomicrographs and Summary Results of Bulk Sample and Fiber Analysis

New cut-resistant sleeve

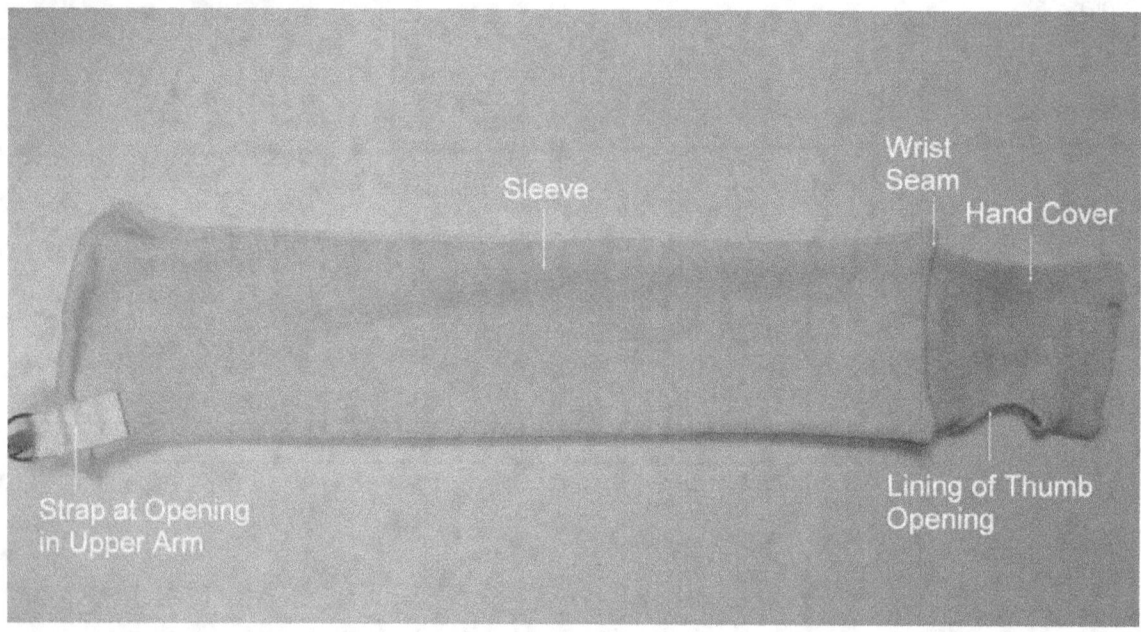

Figure C1. Photomicrograph showing outside of new sleeve.

Laundered cut-resistant sleeve

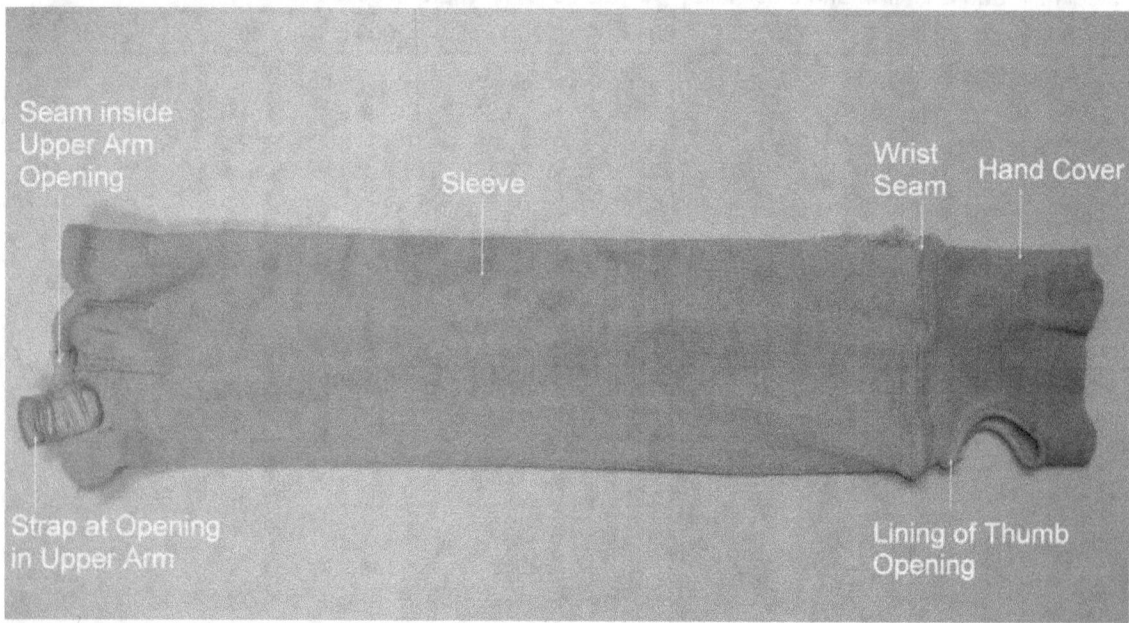

Figure C2. Photomicrograph showing outside of laundered sleeve.

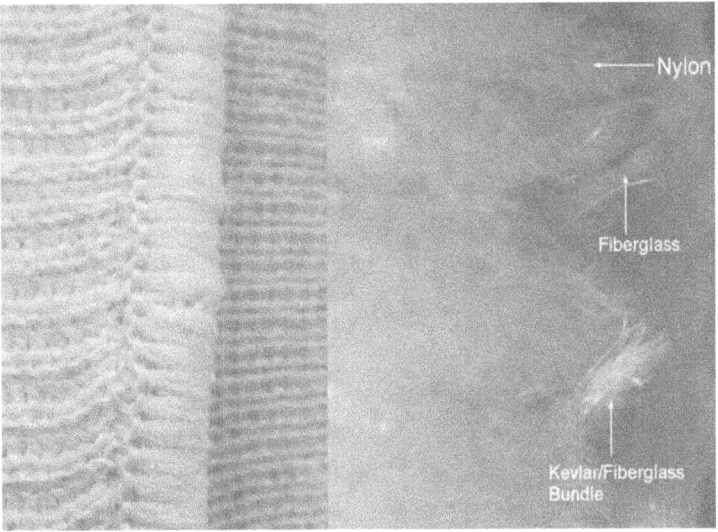

Figure C3. Photomicrographs showing wrist seam. RIGHT: Showing Kevlar and fiberglass coming through nylon at 20X.

New sleeve wrist seam

The yellow seam at the wrist was composed of nylon and joined the sleeve and hand cover materials from the inside. Even though the seam did not show signs of wear, Kevlar and broken fiberglass bundles were observed coming through the seam (Figure C3).

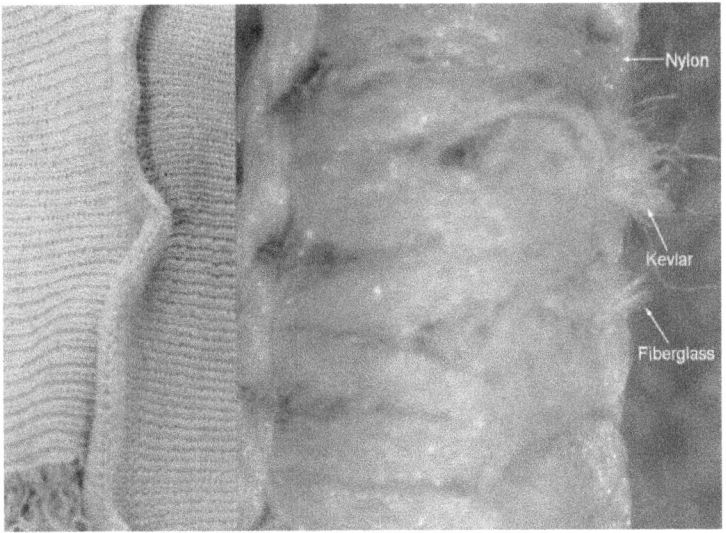

Figure C4. Photomicrographs showing a laundered wrist seam. RIGHT: Showing Kevlar and broken fiberglass bundles coming through nylon seam at 20X.

Laundered sleeve wrist seam

This seam was composed of nylon and joined the sleeve and hand cover materials from the inside. The seam was worn down, and the nylon bundles were frayed. Kevlar and fiberglass from the sleeve and hand cover were coming through the seam where it was worn down (Figure C4). No fiberglass was observed in one of the samples.

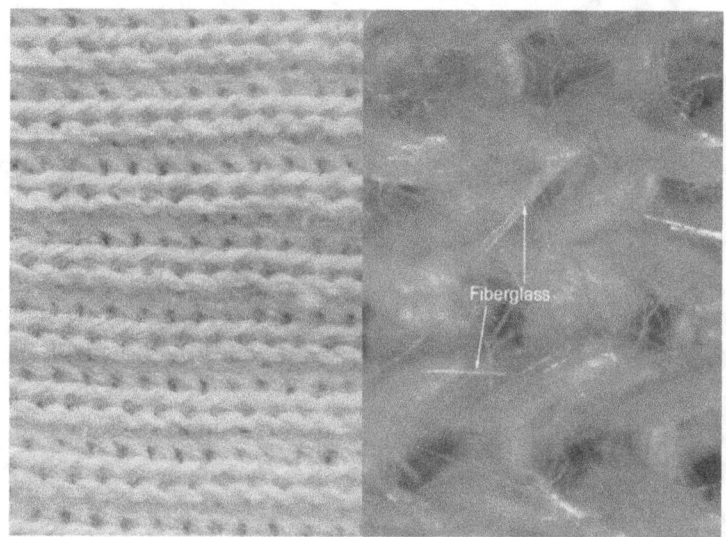

Figure C5. Photomicrographs showing a new sleeve. RIGHT: Showing broken fiberglass bundles at 20X.

New sleeve

The new sleeve was composed of fiberglass and Kevlar bundles woven together. The material did not show signs of wear or tearing. Individual fibers and broken bundles of fiberglass were observed protruding from both the outside and inside of the sleeve (Figure C5). Blue cellulose fibers were stuck to the inside surface of the material of two of the samples.

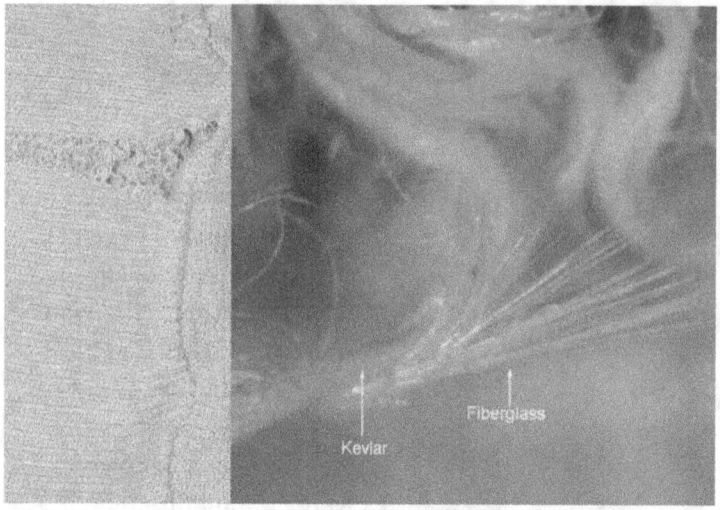

Figure C6. Photomicrographs showing tear in sleeve. RIGHT: Showing broken fiberglass bundles in tear at 15X.

Laundered sleeve

The laundered sleeve was composed of fiberglass and Kevlar bundles woven together. On the inside and outside of the sleeve, where the material did not appear to be torn, individual fibers and broken fiberglass bundles were observed protruding from the sleeve. In the areas where the material was torn (Figure C6), the Kevlar bundles appeared to be frayed. Blue cellulose fibers were stuck to the inside surface of the material in one of the samples. Gray paint was observed on one sleeve sample.

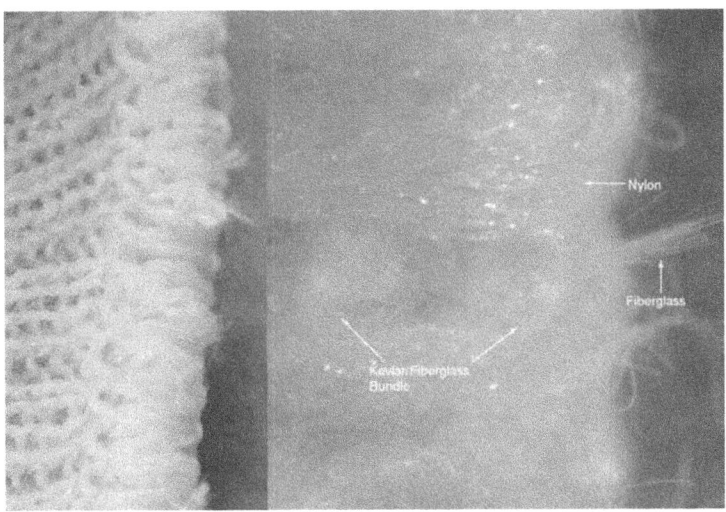

Figure C7. Photomicrographs showing seam inside upper arm opening. RIGHT: Showing Kevlar and fiberglass coming through nylon at 20X.

New seam inside upper arm opening

This seam was composed of nylon, and joined the sleeve and cuff materials. Even though the seam was not exposed and did not show signs of wear, Kevlar and broken fiberglass bundles were coming through the seam from the sleeve (Figure C7). Blue cellulose fibers were also observed in one of the samples.

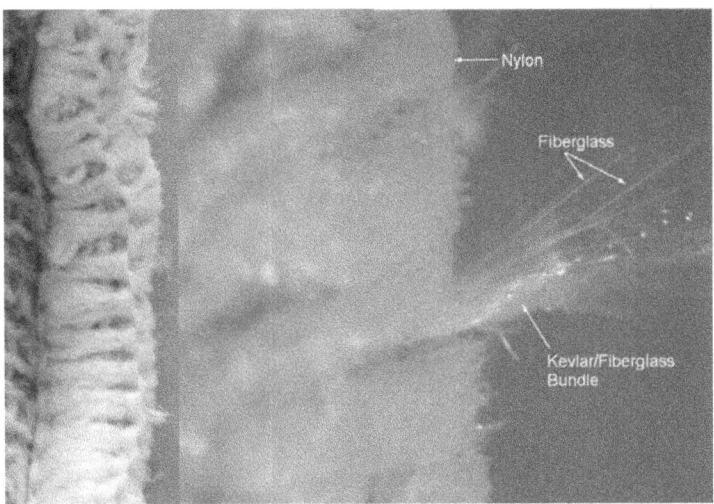

Figure C8. Photomicrographs showing seam inside upper arm opening. RIGHT: Showing Kevlar and fiberglass coming through nylon at 20X.

Laundered seam inside upper arm opening

The yellow seam inside the upper arm opening was composed of nylon and joined the sleeve and cuff materials together. The seam was only exposed in areas where the sleeve had been torn. Kevlar and fiberglass from the sleeve were coming through the seam from the sleeve and cuff materials (Figure C8).

Fibers from cut-resistant sleeve

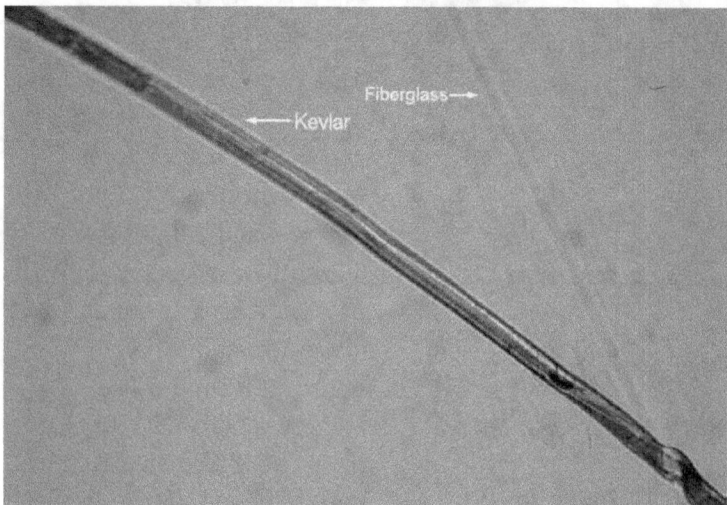

Figure C9. Photomicrograph showing Kevlar and fiberglass from sleeve.

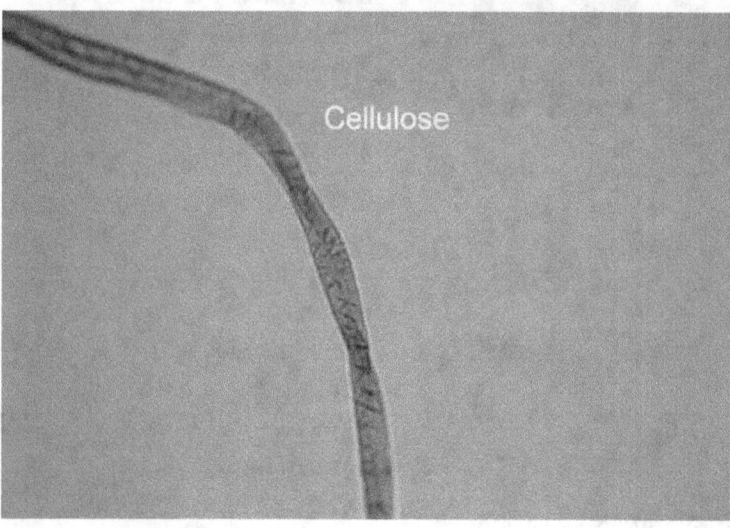

Figure C10. Photomicrograph showing cellulose from sleeve.

Yellow insulation

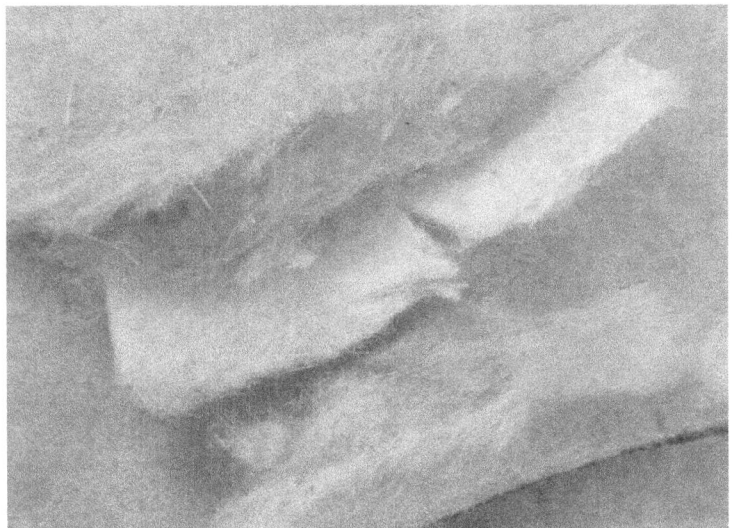

Figure C11. Photomicrograph of yellow insulation.

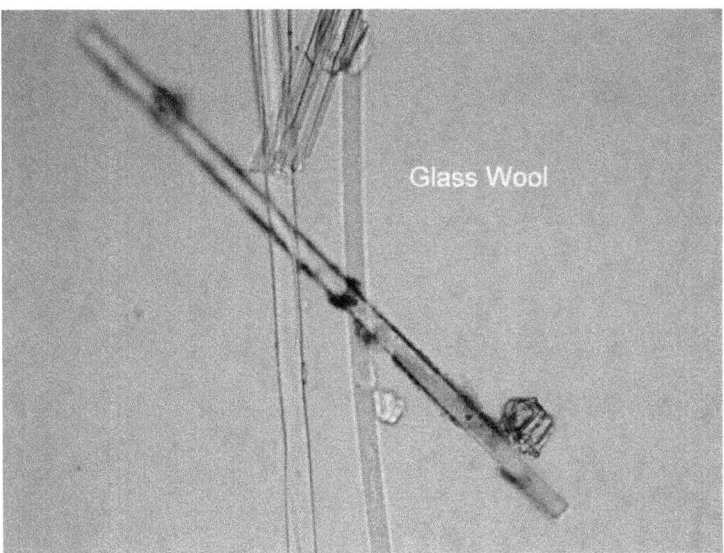

Figure C12. Photomicrograph of glass wool from yellow insulation.

White fibrous material

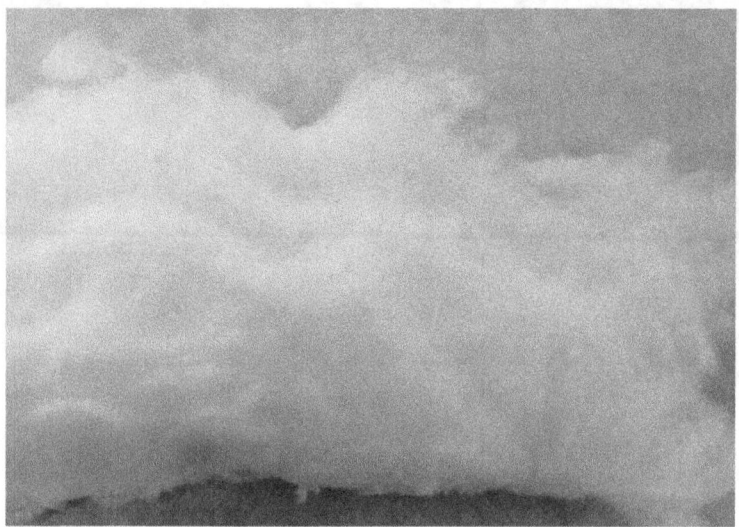

Figure C13. Photomicrograph of white Kaowool.

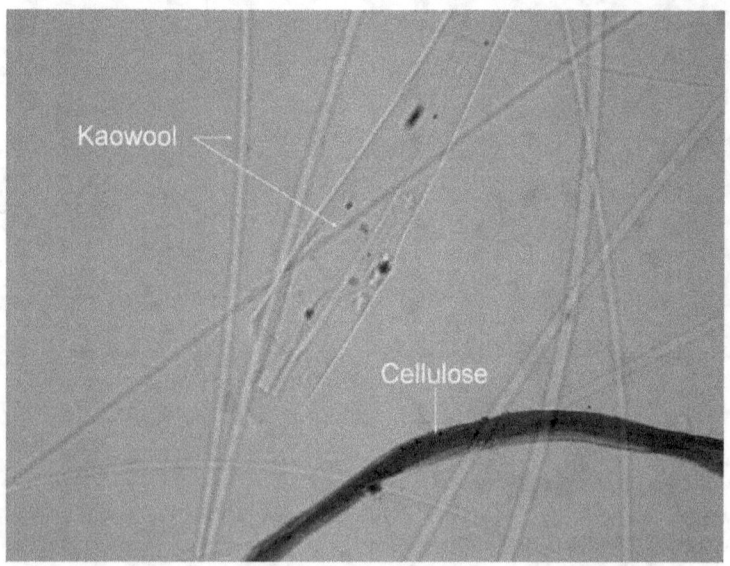

Figure C14. Photomicrograph of Kaowool and cellulose from white fibrous material.

Appendix D: Health Effects

Fiberglass

Fiberglass is a manmade fiber also known as fibrous glass or glass fibers. These fibers are used to insulate and protect products from impact and high temperatures. Fiberglass is made by pulling molten glass through small holes. These filaments can be made short (glass wool fibers) or long (continuous filament glass fibers). Short fibers are used to make insulation commonly used in residential buildings. The continuous filaments can be twisted together to form yarn, such as E-glass, that can be woven into a fiberglass fabric or with other materials into fabrics with desired properties. Some workplace protective sleeves containing E-glass fibers are used to protect employees from heat and lacerations.

Exposure to glass fibers may cause eye, respiratory, and skin irritation. Glass fibers of widths > 3.5 µm are known to cause dermatitis from mechanical skin irritation, which is characterized by itching or prickling, especially in skin folds. For most workers, symptoms disappear within a week or two of exposure, but they may persist in some individuals. Allergic contact dermatitis may occur from exposure to the resins used in the fiberglass products [Adams 1999]. Large width fibers (> 3.5 µm) are also responsible for irritation of the eyes and upper respiratory tract, whereas smaller width fibers (< 3 µm) can enter gas exchange regions of the lung [ATSDR 2002; ACGIH 2012].

The dimensions, durability, and dose of glass fibers determine their toxicity [Cullen et al. 2000; NTP 2011]. Generally, any fibers that are < 3.5 µm in width may deposit deep in the lung and are called "respirable" fibers [WHO 2000; EPA 2001]. Depending on their length and composition, these small fibers may be cleared from the lung by dissolution or by macrophage destruction or translocation [Hesterberg and Hart 2001]. If the body is unable to clear these fibers, chronic inflammation and fibrosis may occur, and over time there is an increased risk of lung disease and cancer formation. One well-known example of this is the risk of lung disease and cancer from asbestos. Inhaled fibers of greater widths are deposited primarily in the upper airways (mouth, nose, throat), where they are more readily removed by the clearance mechanisms of the respiratory tract.

E-glass fibers are made in a range of widths, generally between 3 µm and 20 µm [Wallenberger et al. 2001]. Most have a width greater than 3.5 µm and are inhalable, but not respirable [IARC 2002]. Crushing, chopping, or other mechanical processing such as washing may break glass fibers horizontally, making them shorter, but because glass fibers do not break longitudinally, they do not become smaller in width. The 2011 National Toxicology Program Report on Carcinogens states that certain glass wool fibers that are inhalable are reasonably anticipated to be human carcinogens on the basis of animal studies and studies of fiber durability (i.e., fibers that are biopersistent in the lung or tracheobronchial region) [NTP 2011]. The certain glass fibers they refer to have widths less than 3 µm and include ingredients that make the fibers difficult to dissolve or break apart. No evidence of an increased risk of respiratory disease or death due to glass fiber exposure has been found among studies of fiberglass manufacturing workers in Europe, Canada, and the United States [Hesterberg and Hart 2001].

The NIOSH recommended exposure limit (REL) for fiberglass in air is 5 mg/m³ (total particulate) as an 8-hour time-weighted average (TWA), with a limit of 3 fibers per cubic centimeter of air for fibers ≤ 3.5 μm in width, and ≥ 10 μm in length. The REL is based on increased health concern of fibrosis and respiratory tract irritation in longer, small width fibers [NIOSH 1988].

The OSHA permissible exposure limit (PEL) for fiberglass dust in air is 15 mg/m³ (total particulate) and 5 mg/m³ for the respirable fraction, determined as 8-hour averages [OSHA 2006]. The American Conference of Governmental Industrial Hygienists (ACGIH) threshold limit value (TLV) for exposure to continuous-filament glass fibers, glass wool fibers, and special purpose glass fibers is 1 fiber per cubic centimeter of air for fibers > 5 μm in length and < 3 μm in width, with an aspect ratio > 5:1 (length to width). In addition, the ACGIH recommends that exposure to the inhalable fraction of continuous filament glass fibers not exceed 5 mg/m³. The critical effect, which is the basis for the TLV, is irritation [ACGIH 2012].

Para-Aramid Fibers (Kevlar Fibers)

Para-aramid fibers are manufactured from long chain synthetic polyamide and are spun into yarn and fabrics or incorporated into composites. The fibers have a high strength-to-weight ratio, heat resistance, and chemical resistance. Typical para-aramid fibers are 12–15 microns in diameter, but during processing, fibrils of < 1 micron diameter can break off the core fiber and become airborne [IARC 1997]. Several studies of animals exposed to airborne para-aramid fibrils have found that, unlike asbestos fibers, the para-aramid fibrils deposited in the lungs of the animals are broken down into even smaller fibrils that are more easily cleared from the body. Para-aramid fibrils have not been shown to cause chronic disease; however, no human data are available regarding Kevlar fibril exposure [Lockey 1996; IARC 1997]. The World Health Organization's International Agency for Research on Cancer (IARC) has concluded that there is inadequate evidence of para-aramid fibril exposure causing cancer in humans [IARC 1997].

Sampling methods used for these fibers are similar to those used for inorganic fibers such as asbestos or man-made mineral fibers. During manufacturing and end use, airborne fibril levels have been reported to range from 0.01 to 0.4 fibers per cubic centimeter for an 8-hour TWA [Lockey 1996]. Although there are no current recommended exposure levels for para-aramid fibrils, fibril concentrations maintained near the level typically found in current commercial operations (0.5 fibers per cubic centimeter or less) are not known to pose a health risk to humans [Lockey 1996].

References

ACGIH [2011]. Synthetic vitreous fibers. In: Documentation of the threshold limit values and biological exposure indices. Cincinnati, OH: American Conference of Government Industrial Hygienists.

ACGIH [2012]. 2012 TLVs® and BEIs®: threshold limit values for chemical substances and physical agents and biological exposure indices. Cincinnati, OH: American Conference of Governmental Industrial Hygienists.

Adams RM [1999]. Dermatitis due to fibrous glass. In: Adams RM, ed. Occupational skin disease, 3rd ed. Philadelphia, PA: W.B. Saunders Company, pp. 11–12.

AM Health and Safety [2011]. Cut-resistant sleeve study by AM Health and Safety (AM H&S) and RJ Lee Group (RJLG), Pittsburgh, PA. Report written on May 27, 2010 by Keith Rickabaugh, Technical director, Materials and Analytical Services, AM H&S.

ASTM [1997]. ASTM F1790-97 Standard test method for measuring cut resistance of materials used in protective clothing. West Conshohocken, PA: ASTM International.

ASTM [2005]. ASTM D3389-05 Standard test method for coated fabrics abrasion resistance (Rotary platform abrader). West Conshohocken, PA: ASTM International.

ATSDR [2002]. Technical briefing paper: Health effects from exposure to fibrous glass, rock wool, or slag wool. U.S. Department of Health and Human Services, Agency for Toxic Substances and Disease Registry; Contract No. 205-1999-00024. [http://www.atsdr.cdc.gov/DT/fibrous-glass.html]. Date accessed: May 2013.

BLS [2010]. Bureau of Labor Statistics occupational injuries and illnesses incidence rate calculator and comparison tool webpage [http://data.bls.gov/iirc/]. Tabular data, 2010: total number of nonfatal work-related injury and illness cases, number of cases involving days away from work, and number of cases involving job transfer or restricted work activity only, by industry. Date accessed: May 2013.

Bureau Veritas North America [2000] Scanning electron microscopy/energy dispersive spectroscopy standard operating procedure. Bureau Veritas North America, Inc.

Chang CH, Shih YC [2007]. The effects of glove thickness and work load on female hand performance and fatigue during an infrequent high-intensity gripping task. Appl Ergon *38*(3):317–324.

Cullen RT, Searl A, Buchanan D, Davis JMG, Miller BG, Jones AD [2000]. Pathogenicity of a special-perose glass microfiber (E glass) relative to another glass microfiber and amosite asbestos. Inhalation Toxicol *12*(10):959–977.

Dianat I, Haslegrave CM, Stedmon AW [2012]. Using pliers in assembly work: short and long task duration effects of gloves on hand performance capabilities and subjective assessments of discomfort and ease of tool manipulation. Applied Ergonomics *43*(2):413–423.

EPA [1982]. Environmental monitoring systems laboratory–interim method for the determination of asbestos in bulk insulation samples. Washington DC: U.S. Environmental Protection Agency, Publication No. EPA 600/M4-82-020.

EPA [1993]. Method for the determination of asbestos in bulk building materials (PLM). Washington DC: U.S. Environmental Protection Agency, Publication No. EPA 600/R-93/116.

EPA [2001]. Health effects test guidelines: OPPTS 870.8355 Combined chronic toxicity/carcinogenicity testing of respirable fibrous particles. The Office of Prevention, Pesticides and Toxic Substances, U.S. Environmental Protection Agency. EPA 712–C–01–352. [http://www.regulations.gov/#!documentDetail;D=EPA-HQ-OPPT-2009-0156-0050]. Date accessed: May 2013.

Heisel EB, Hunt FE [1968]. Further studies in cutaneous reactions to glass fibers. Arch Environ Health *17*(5):705–711.

Hesterberg TW, Hart GA [2001]. Synthetic vitreous fibers: a review of toxicology research and its impact on hazard classification. Crit Rev Toxicol *31*(1):1–53.

Hsieh MY, Guo YL, Shiao JSC, Sheu HM [2001]. Morphology of glass fibers in electronics workers with fiberglass dermatitis – a scanning electron microscopy study. Int J Dermatol *40*(4):258–261.

IARC [1997]. IARC monographs on the evaluation of carcinogenic risks to humans: silica, some silicates, coal dust and para-aramid fibrils. Vol. 68. Lyon, France: World Health Organization, International Agency for Research on Cancer.

IARC [2002]. IARC Monographs on the evaluation of carcinogenic risks to humans: man-made vitreous fibres. Vol. 81. Lyon, France: World Health Organization, International Agency for Research on Cancer. pp. 327-339. [http://monographs.iarc.fr/ENG/Monographs/vol81/mono81-6E.pdf]. Date accessed: May 2013.

Kopka A, Crawford JM, Broome IJ [2005]. Anesthetists should wear gloves – touch sensitivity is improved with a new type of thin glove. Acta Anaesthesiol Scand *49*(4):459–462.

Kominsky JR, Millette JR [2010]. Evaluation of asbestos in dust on surfaces by micro-vacuum and wipe sampling. J ASTM Int *8*(5):1–8.

Krause M, Geer W, Swenson L, Fallah P, Robbins C [2006]. Controlled study of mold growth and cleaning procedure on treated and untreated wet gypsum wallboard in an indoor environment. J Occup Environ Hyg *3*(8):435–441.

Laroche C, Barr A, Dong H, Rempel D [2007]. Effect of dental tool surface texture and material on static friction with a wet gloved fingertip. J Biomech *40*(3):697–701.

Lockey JE [1996]. Man-made fibers and nonasbestos fibrous silicates, In: Harber P, Schenker M, Balmes J, eds. Occupational and environmental respiratory disease. Mosby-Year Book, Inc., St. Louis, MO: pp. 330–344.

McCrone WC [1980]. The asbestos particle atlas. Ann Arbor, MI: Ann Arbor Science Publishers, Inc.

NFPA [2006]. Report on Comments A2006: NFPA 1971 Standard on protective ensembles for structural fire fighting and proximity fire fighting. Quincy, MA: National Fire Protection Association [http://www.nfpa.org/assets/files/PDF/ROP/1971-A2006-ROC-Preprint.pdf]. Date accessed: May 2013.

NIOSH [1988]. Testimony to the Department of Labor on the Occupational Safety and Health Administration proposed rule on air contaminants. Washington, D.C.

NIOSH [1997]. Protect your family: reduce contamination at home. U.S. Department of Health and Human Services, Centers for Disease Control and Prevention, National Institute for Occupational Safety and Health, DHHS (NIOSH) Publication Number 97-125. [http://www.cdc.gov/niosh/docs/97-125/]. Date accessed: May 2013.

NIOSH [2013]. NIOSH manual of analytical methods (NMAM®). 4th ed. Schlecht PC, O'Connor PF, eds. Cincinnati, OH: U.S. Department of Health and Human Services, Centers for Disease Control and Prevention, National Institute for Occupational Safety and Health, DHHS (NIOSH) Publication 94–113 (August, 1994); 1st Supplement Publication 96135, 2nd Supplement Publication 98-119; 3rd Supplement 2003-154. [http://www.cdc.gov/niosh/docs/2003-154/]. Date accessed: May 2013.

NTP [2011]. Certain glass wool fibers (inhalable). In: Report on carcinogens. 12th ed. U.S. Department of Human and Health Services, National Toxicology Program. Research Triangle Park, NC. [http://ntp.niehs.nih.gov/ntp/roc/twelfth/profiles/GlassWoolFibers.pdf]. Date accessed: May 2013.

OSHA [2006]. Fibrous glass dust: chemical sampling information. Occupational Safety and Health Administration. [http://www.osha.gov/dts/chemicalsampling/data/CH_242120.html]. Date accessed: May 2013.

Possick PA, Gellin GA, Key MM [1970]. Fibrous glass dermatitis. Am Ind Hyg Assn J *31*(1):12–15.

Salonen HJ, Lappalainen SK, Riuttala HM, Tossavainen AP, Pasanen PO, Reijula KE [2009]. Man-made vitreous fibers in office buildings in the Helsinki area. J Occup Environ Hyg *6*(10):624–631.

SKC, Inc. [2011]. Stick-to-it operating instructions, form #40065 Rev 1102. [http://www.skcinc.com/instructions/40065.pdf]. Date accessed: May 2013.

Urzì C, De Leo F [2001]. Sampling with adhesive tape strips: an easy and rapid method to monitor microbial colonization on monument surfaces. J Microbiol Methods *44*(1):1–11.

Wallenberger FT, Watson JC, Li H [2001]. Glass fibers. In: Miracle DB, Donaldson SL, eds. ASM Handbook. Vol. 21: Composites. Materials Park, Ohio: ASM International, pp. 27–34.

Waters TR, Putz-Anderson V, Garg A [1994]. Applications manual for the revised NIOSH lifting equation. Cincinnati, OH: Centers for Disease Control and Prevention, National Institute for Occupational Safety and Health, DHHS (NIOSH) Publication 94-110.

WHO [2000]. Air quality guidelines for Europe. 2nd ed. European series. No. 91. Copenhagen, Denmark: World Health Organization. [http://www.euro.who.int/__data/assets/pdf_file/0005/74732/E71922.pdf]. Date accessed: May 2013.

Wimer B, McDowell TW, Xu XS, Welcome DE, Warren C, Dong RG [2010]. Effects of gloves on the total grip strength applied to cylindrical handles. Intl J Industrial Ergon *40*(5):574–583.

Keywords: NAICS 331111 (Iron and Steel Mills), steel production, fiberglass, skin irritation, respiratory irritation, protective sleeves

The Health Hazard Evaluation Program investigates possible health hazards in the workplace under the authority of Section 20(a)(6) of the Occupational Safety and Health Act of 1970, 29 U.S.C. 669(a)(6). The Health Hazard Evaluation Program also provides, upon request, technical assistance to federal, state, and local agencies to control occupational health hazards and to prevent occupational illness and disease. Regulations guiding the Program can be found in Title 42, Code of Federal Regulations, Part 85; Requests for Health Hazard Evaluations (42 CFR 85).

Acknowledgments

Analytical Support: Tiffany Dixon, Bureau Veritas North America
Desktop Publishers: Greg Hartle and Mary Winfree
Editor: Ellen Galloway
Ergonomic Assistance: Jessica Ramsey
Health Communicator: Stefanie Brown
Industrial Hygiene Field Assistance: Greg Burr
Literature Review Assistance: Dorathy Lachman
Logistics: Donnie Booher and Karl Feldmann
Medical Field Assistance: Francisco Meza

Availability of Report

Recommended citation for this report:
NIOSH [2013]. Health hazard evaluation report: evaluation of cut-resistant sleeves and fiberglass fiber shedding at a steel mill. By Tapp L, Ceballos D, Wiegand D. Cincinnati, OH: U.S. Department of Health and Human Services, Centers for Disease Control and Prevention, National Institute for Occupational Safety and Health, NIOSH HETA No. 2011-0113-3179.

To receive NIOSH documents or more information about occupational safety and health topics, please contact NIOSH:

> Telephone: 1–800–CDC–INFO (1–800–232–4636)
>
> TTY: 1–888–232–6348
>
> CDC INFO: www.cdc.gov/info
>
> or visit the NIOSH Web site at www.cdc.gov/niosh
>
> For a monthly update on news at NIOSH, subscribe to NIOSH eNews by visiting www.cdc.gov/niosh/eNews.

SAFER • HEALTHIER • PEOPLE™